Magical Healing

How to Use Your Mind to Heal Yourself and Others

GW00468897

Angela Kaelin

2013
Winter Tempest Books

ISBN: 0615739938
ISBN-13: 978-0615739939
Winter Tempest Books

DEDICATION

In honor of my grandparents.

CONTENTS

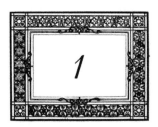

ABOUT MAGICAL HEALING

This book is a plain, simple, practical presentation of a system of magical healing wherein the term, "magic," represents an esoteric science. This advanced, ancient science stands in contradiction to the official science of the state, which is of a materialist nature.

While magic is sometimes an element in religion, it is not, itself, a religion. Anyone, regardless of their faith or lack thereof, can perform magical healing by closely following the instructions in this book.

The magic of healing is based on natural laws. It is the effect of the manipulation of subtle forces, which are a natural part of our physical environment. This energy has been given different names by different occultists and scientists of different backgrounds at different times, including the terms: Vital force; life energy; animal magnetism or the magnetic fluid; Odic force; orgone; prana and chi, just to name a few. This energy is more or less fine at different levels or frequencies and it animates and imparts a kind of intelligence to all things in the world most of us perceive with our five senses, as well things in the worlds beyond.

When this energy can be perceived in human beings through the hands and seen radiating from the body, it is commonly called the aura. This energy can be magnified and manipulated to heal the chakra system as well as organs and systems of the physical body.

Some aspects of magical healing are similar to Reiki, a popular healing system founded in Japan in 1922 by Dr. Mikao Usu. But, it is not Reiki. Furthermore, you do not need to belong to a group, receive any special symbols or receive a "degree" from any master. You are already a master. You only need to learn how to increase and direct the natural forces that run through your body and throughout the cosmos.

You will master magical healing by doing it and proving to yourself that it works. You can, also, safely use these techniques to heal other people and animals. Since you do not have to make contact with or, in fact, even be in the same room with another person to effect this healing, there is no problem with medical liability. Although, it is always legally prudent to give the advisory that one should seek allopathic medical treatment when you are doing work for another person. In the case of emergency some of these techniques (such as techniques to stop bleeding) can be used after you have called for medical services and you are waiting for the ambulance to arrive.

This book is not intended to instruct in the treatment or diagnosis of diseases. Rather, it is a course in the manipulation of magical energies which rests upon the foundation of a number of esoteric philosophies and practices – some from the East and some from the West. Magic and healing are universal concepts, which are used with the intention of keeping the body completely healthy. It works on principles completely contrary to the philosophy of modern medicine and the two should not be confused.

The reader who applies the information in this book should be able to do things that appear miraculous to some. People are amazed when you can wave your hands in the air and take away their pain. But, it is here I want to caution you. It is my hope that you will share what you know about healing with other people and not let your ego get the best of you.

There are not enough healers in the world to heal all of the sickness, so it is important for us to be self-healers and to teach what we know to anyone who will listen.

Please, study the material in this book and then choose which aspects appeal to you most and put these into practice first. If you are familiar with other systems of healing, you can incorporate what you already know into the methods described. Other systems might include nutritional therapy, herbalism, homeopathy, acupuncture (or acupressure) and reflexology all of which incorporate elements of magical healing because all involve the promotion of the life force.

Apart from being able to heal yourself and others without touching them, without the use of any substance or agent and even at great distances, there are other benefits to learning these techniques.

Learning how to use the science and art of magical healing will increase your ability to perform other types of magic like divination, spell casting and black or white magic because of the similar skills required, such as visualization, establishing resonance with a subject and the application of the will.

Some people bristle at the idea of black magic because the esoteric science of magic on its most fundamental level knows no nuances of color. Energy will obey the commands of the magician whether his intentions are good or evil and whether he is pure or impure. Many magicians around the world perform both black and white magic proficiently without making hypocritical judgments. Healers are often sought after, but, also, feared in cultures where this principle is understood because the people know that the power to heal is no different from the power to harm.

As you proceed through this book, you will see how the techniques presented can be used to increase your power and efficacy in all magical practices so that you become a channel for the life force which permeates all things both animate and inanimate.

It is important to not only read this book, but to put the exercises into practice along with the visualizations. As you read, make the physical motions described in *Chapter 4* until they become natural and add the visualizations to these motions until it becomes automatic. These are the most fundamental aspects of learning magical healing.

2

THE POWER OF THE MIND AND BODY

The power of the mind is the power of the will. Most people agree that the mind is powerful and that it has the power to help the body heal itself. What most of them do not understand is how to use their minds to do this, otherwise, more people would be doing it and there would be far less ill-health in the world.

If you want to be a healer, you must begin with the physical foundation of good health. Without it, your body and every cell in it will become weak and the energetic connectivity will slow down. With this physical weakness comes a mental weakness that eventually renders the mind unable to assert and direct its will upon the energetic currents.

To support the mind with a healthy body, you need: Exercise, good nutrition, hydration, oxygenation and a large personal supply of life energy or vital force.

Exercise may include some mild cardiovascular health-promoting activity like walking, swimming, dancing or rebounding (jumping on a trampoline which is excellent for lymphatic system function) and many people find great benefits in bodybuilding, isometric exercises or Pilate's.

The question of proper nutrition is considerably more clouded because of government recommendations which are usually incomplete or inadequate.

A more simple, if not primitive, diet of unprocessed food and broth made from the bones and ligaments of fish, cattle and poultry help give the body's tissues what they need to grow and repair themselves. This is contrary to the recommendations of most Western physicians, but it has been the recommendation of many objective nutritional researchers.

Because of the depletion and contamination of our soil due to modern farming methods which employ poisons, it is considered wise to supplement your diet with vitamins and minerals, including trace minerals.

As a result of events involving the reactor core of the Fukushima nuclear power plant in Japan in the aftermath of the earthquakes and subsequent tsunami of March 2011, more people have recognized the need for supplements to offset the decaying effects of radioactive isotopes. Nutritional experts recommend seaweed for its natural supply of iodine (a natural trace mineral, which should not be confused with iodide) or a seaweed supplement like Sea-Adine by Heritage Products, taken once a day to help the body absorb the good healthful trace minerals and make them part of your tissues instead of absorbing cancer-causing radioactive isotopes. Some experts further recommend other dietary supplements such as L-Glutamine (glutamic acid), MSM (methyl sulfonyl methane), blue green algae (spirulina) and chlorella as well as other chelators to combat the destructive effects of other elements in radiation poisoning such as cesium and plutonium.

Processed foods and those containing preservatives and additives should be avoided as much as possible in favor of whole, raw foods.

One of the healthiest ways to supply nutrition to the body is through the juicing of raw foods, which contain live enzymes. This living food enhances the body's supply of vital energy. By contrast, eating cooked, pasteurized, dead food, which is devoid of such energy-supplying enzymes, depletes the body's supply of life force energy by causing it to work harder to process it.

Proper hydration is necessary to promote the electro-conductivity of the vital force and facilitate its purification, a good supply of clean, uncontaminated water should be consumed every day. Distilled water may prove to be the best choice, at this time, because of environmental concerns and the difficulty of filtering very tiny particles.

Oxygenation of all the cells in the body is accomplished through the proper breathing technique. Most people in the western world do not breathe deeply enough because of constrictive clothing and stress.

The breath is the life. This is a very old belief in the western tradition as well as the eastern one. With the first breath people enter the living world and with their last breath they leave it. The breath is traditionally believed to contain the spirit and when people die, it is said they "give up the ghost."

Proper inhalation delivers a fresh supply of healthy vital energy while exhalation cleans out old, dirty, depleted energy. Most of us must re-learn to breathe properly, this involves a process of using the conscious mind to re-train the unconscious mind. It results in clearer thinking and greater vitality.

Through all of the aforementioned methods and by the power of the will, you must cultivate a large personal supply of the vital force to be a healthy, powerful and highly effective magical healer.

Cell and Organ Intelligence

Esoteric science teaches that the mind is comprised of different levels of consciousness. Some functions are coordinated instinctively, such as digestion, elimination and the healing of the skin after it has been cut. This work is done without the conscious direction of the mind.

It is done because each cell and each organ of the body has a kind of intelligence of its own. Organs "know" how to perform their function and each cell that is part of an organ has a group intelligence. Under normal circumstances the cells and organs know their particular function and they do it without direction from the conscious mind.

But, when they are not functioning properly, a healer can speak to and direct the function of the cells and they will obey, thus restoring the organ to its normal state. And, conversely, the organs and cells can communicate with the healer and impart information about the degree of dysfunction and the method of remedying it.

This is true for every cell of the body and includes the cells of the bones and teeth, which are tissues like any other in the body.

Each cell is separate and independent from the others, just as members of an organization are separate individuals, although they work for a common purpose. When it is functioning properly, each cell works constantly, performing its task of absorbing oxygen and nutrients and throwing off toxic waste. Healthy cells are strong and flexible. They repel attacks from bacterial, fungi and viruses easily. The cells work to grow, repair and eventually replace themselves with fresh, healthy ones.

Cells in the body comprise the teeth, bones, brain, eyes, skin, heart, liver, blood and literally every organ or tissue in the body. Functions are directed and coordinated by the endocrine system, which control the metabolic function, the release of hormones and secretions of the glands. These functions can, also, be directed by the healer.

The Causes of Disease

Surprisingly, even in supposedly advanced western cultures, the foundational cause of disease is malnutrition. With proper nutrition, most adverse health conditions can be thwarted or overcome.

A major secondary cause of disease is the buildup of toxins from pesticides and toxic metals in the system.

There is, also, the problem of drugs – both illicit and prescription. Many of these substances have dangerous side-effects and act as a poison to the body and mind.

Vaccinations have become increasingly controversial as more people awaken to the lack of scientific support for their efficacy and their debilitating and deadly side effects. Childhood vaccines may be the cause of a litany diseases including cancer, Chron's Disease, autism, ADHD, nerve disorders by many names and narcolepsy.

Stress is frequently cited as the number one killer of men and women. It is a silent killer that leads to the two major causes of death: Cardiovascular disease and cancer. Chronic stress depletes the body of vital nutrition, interferes with digestion, respiration, heart function, the release of hormones and the function of the glandular system. It, also, aggravates existing conditions of poor health.

Proper nutrition or what is sometimes called "nutritional therapy" can help remedy many of these problems by giving the body the support it needs to repair and detoxify itself. When the body has the nutrition it needs, it very often heals itself.

These ideas are in contradiction to the fundamental view of conventional medicine which is rooted in the germ theory of Pasteur and carried on by the likes of Lister and Salk. Their philosophical descendants, modern allopathic doctors, believe that diseases are caused by harmful microorganisms.

This is only partially true, of course, because the foundational cause of disease is a weakness in the cells caused by poor nutrition; inadequate elimination of toxins, pesticides and harmful residues; the effects of allopathic medical practices (radiation, vaccination, unnecessary surgeries, drugging and chemotherapy) and stress. These cause the cells of the body to lose their vital force and render the cells, organs and systems of the body unable to defend themselves.

The conventional allopathic remedy to what they perceive as the cause of disease is to kill the offending organisms and destroy diseased tissues. They try to destroy harmful pathogens with their chemical poisons, knives and needles. If they kill healthy cells or remove vital organs from the body, they consider this all part of the process of fighting disease.

By contrast, healers work to strengthen the body and increase its vital force through nutrition and other means of supplying the vital force. Magical healing does this by using the mind to direct the will upon the cells, organs and bodily systems.

3

THE BASIC METHOD OF MAGICAL HEALING

Franz Anton Mesmer, whose methods were misunderstood in his own day, at least, as much as they are now, spoke correctly when he described the energetic force that flows throughout the universe, animating all life, as a "magnetic fluid." When it is viewed by a psychic healer, it appears as a fluid stream or cloud of energy often tinged with different iridescent hues similar to the appearance of the colors in a rainbow.

It has a magnetoelectric quality and can be funneled or directed into cells, organs or chakras or it can be pulled out. In cases where the cells or chakras are depleted of energy, they can be re-energized by the application of this magnetic fluid. And, when there is congestion or when the energy of the body or its system is toxic and depleted, it can be extracted. Whereupon, it is usually replaced with fresh healthy magnetic fluid.

The organs of the body and the chakra centers all have a dual nature. They have polarities just like batteries or magnets do. They can be treated with negative or positive energy flow from the healer and they can be accessed from the front or back of the body.

The chakra system contains many colorful, swirling energy centers. In the eastern system there are seven major chakras that most people are familiar with and a number of powerful minor chakras, which are less familiar.

Each chakra governs the flow of vital energy into different organs and systems of the body and each one has a relationship to the others. The healer should be familiar with the major and some minor chakra centers, as follows:

Base or Root Chakra: The base of spine, legs, bones, feet, rectum and immune system. This center is located at the perineum. Its colors are dark red, dark orange and a little golden yellow.

Sacral or Sex Chakra: The sexual organs, large intestines, lower vertebrae, pelvis, appendix, bladder and hips. This center is located at the tailbone. Its main color is orange.

Navel Chakra: The lower intestines, appendix, adrenal glands and energy flow. The Navel chakra is the key to energy flow into the body. When it is accessed from the back it can be used to tweak the energy level, but it should not be manipulated on infants and pregnant women. Its color is mostly golden yellow with some dark red. (This is a separate center from the Solar Plexus and the Spleen chakras, but some systems regard the three centers as one because they are very closely related.)

Spleen Chakra: It is the entry point for the flow of life energy into the body. It is located in the left side of the body at about the second rib and is mid-way between the Navel and Solar Plexus chakras. It is a mixture of all colors.

Solar Plexus: Abdomen, stomach, upper intestines, liver, gall bladder, kidneys, pancreas and adrenal glands. This center is located at about the top of the stomach between the opening in the rib cage. Its colors are yellow, orange and red.

Heart Chakra: The heart and circulatory system, lungs, shoulders and arms, ribs, breasts, diaphragm and thymus gland. This center is located at the heart. It is delicate and is most safely accessed from the back of the body, rather than the front. Its color is golden yellow with a little red.

Throat Chakra: Throat, thyroid, trachea, neck vertebrae, mouth, esophagus, parathyroid and hypothalamus. It is located at the hollow of the throat. Its colors are blue and green with a little violet.

Third Eye Chakra: Brain, nervous system, eyes, ears, nose, pineal and pituitary glands. It is located at the center of the forehead. Its primary colors are violet, blue and little green.

Crown Chakra: Muscular system, skeletal system and skin. It is located on the center of the top of the head. Its colors are violet, blue and white with a small mixture of other colors.

This energy of the chakras swirls in a circular pattern, just as water going down a drain swirls according to the polarity of the planet in either hemisphere.

When the chakras centers are all balanced and working properly, they naturally perform the function of taking in and expelling energy without conscious direction. But, during the course of healing, the energy is pulled from the atmosphere and manipulated by the power of the mind. A healer requires an ample supply of personal vital force, as well as a constant awareness of being a channel for this energy during the course of a healing procedure.

A magical healer is, essentially, a witch doctor who can heal by the power of energies and intelligences. He or she moves her hands in circular motions around, up and down the body without making contact. Although, a practiced healer does not need to move his or her hands, but can effect the same healing on his or herself or on another person at a distance solely by the power of the mind. But, in order to achieve this level of skill, it is important to start out with the basics, healing people who are physically present and moving one's hands about in the process, however, this only facilitates the psychic connection.

The healer can determine where there are deficiencies in vital energies of the body, either through psychic vision or by sensing with the hands. If you can see auras and are able to detect over-functioning or under-functioning chakras by this method, then you should use it. Energize major chakras that are under-functioning, manipulate these vortices so that their proper energetic spin is restored.

Some people can visually detect the physical symptoms of certain disorders. For example, a hump placed high on the back can be a sign of a problem with the kidneys and sometimes the face sometimes take on a strangely bloated appearance in the days and weeks preceding a heart attack. By means of magical healing, such organs and their related systems may be revitalized and restored.

Emotional and mental disturbances in people can, also, be remedied through magical healing. People who have entity attachments or are the victims of psychic attack or psychic vampirism can be freed and healed by directing this magnetic fluid and cutting the cords, which are emotionally draining or adversely influencing the person.

Exercise to Sense the Auric Field

While not everyone has a highly developed ability to see auras or recognize possible signs of disease, almost everyone can sense areas of energetic depletion using their hands. To do this, you must first become aware of this vital energy in the palms of your hands. It has negative and positive polarities and so does your body. Your right hand has a positive charge and your left hand has a negative charge.

Test the energy radiating from your palms. Rub your hands together vigorously for the count of 10. Then, pull them about two feet apart, fingers slightly open, palms facing each other with your thumbs up. Let yourself be aware of this static-like electricity in your hands as you slowly move them together. Let your hands be drawn together until the point where you feel an energetic resistance pushing out, radiating out from one palm to the other. At this point, you could continue to push your hands entirely together if you wanted to, but you feel this resistance pulling them apart.

Repeat this exercise until you become fully aware of this energy. You can, also, use this exercise to activate your awareness of this energy flowing through your hands preceding a healing session.

Now, run your hands over parts of your own or some

willing subject's body. Note at what distance from the body you sense the auric field radiating outward. A healthy body will have energy radiating from every part of the body at a fairly consistent distance outward. An energy field of 3 to 5 inches is normal. Anything less than around 2 inches is a sign of low vitality, depleted energy and illness.

Energy depletion may be detected in the auric field two to three days before symptoms of the illness strike. This is often true in the cases of the common cold and the flu.

The main supply of vital energy the healer works with is obtained from the air through the drawing of the breath and through the chakras and magnified by the healer's mind. It can be transmitted through the breath and the gaze. And, it can also be channeled and magnified through magical tools such as wands, crystals and crystal balls.

4

MAGICAL HEALING IN PRACTICE

The way to begin the practice of magical healing is through the use of the hands. After you have mastered this, you can move on to entirely mental and other methods.

While you can perform magical healing on yourself, for your first experiments, enlist the help of a cooperative and open-minded friend.

Exercise #1: Begin by making passes over the body. Have your friend seat himself on a stool, lie down or stand as he wishes.

Hold your hands several inches apart, with your fingers extended and separated. Raise your hands above his head and bring them downward slowly in a sweeping motion down to his knees. When the pass is completed, flick your fingers as if you were throwing water from them to eliminate any depleted or excess energy.

Visualize this energy being destroyed in flames as you do this.

Then, bring your hands up slowly along the sides of the patient, with your palms down and fingers close together. Then, once again make a sweeping motion with your palms facing outward toward your subject and your fingers separated. This time, sweep down with each of your hands a little further out than before so that you are sweeping a new section of his energetic field. Again, release the depleted or excess energy with a flick of your fingers and see it consumed in flames.

Repeat these motions a number of times until they become familiar and natural to you.

Then, add the following visualization:

Close your eyes and visualize laser-like beams of light extending from your palms and fingertips. When you open your eyes, continue to see this vision of a stream of light, tinged with a slightly blue hue, flowing from your hands and fingers.

If you have difficulty with this visualization, take a laser pointer or small flash light in hand and position its beam so that it appears to be emitting from your palms and fingers. This is the image you must hold in your mind when you are energizing the body. The most important thing is that you see this energy coming from your hands and fingers. As you practice, reality will follow what at first seems to be only imagination.

Practice with this visualization and long sweeping motion until it becomes second nature. Now, when you move your hands and fingers in an energizing motion and sweep, you always see this energetic beam of light flowing from your palms and fingers. Allow yourself to feel the flow of this energy.

This method of sweeping the energy helps to properly

distribute the body's vital force.

Moving the energy in long downward strokes like this will have a relaxing effect on your friend. When you have finished your first practice session, you may want to re-energize him by pouring some vital energy from your fingertips in a light upward motion. Three or four very short upward motions of the hand are sufficient.

When you begin a healing session, start by doing a series of these gentle, long, sweeping strokes before proceeding to other types of motions.

Healing motions should always be made in a downward sweep – never an upward one, except in the case of the brief, gentle re-energizing described above. Your fingers must be spread out and extended to their full length when you energize. When you return your hands to the patient's head for the next sweeping pass, your upward movements must be made along the sides of the patient, with fingers closed and palms turned downward.

No special distance from the body should be maintained, let your intuition be your guide in this matter. As you practice these movements, you will learn the correct distance. But, it is never necessary to touch another person because the laser-like beams of light from your palms and fingertips will make the necessary energetic connection.

In general, slower movements with long strokes of the hands tend to produce a sense of relaxation, rest and relief. More rapid movements with shorter strokes have a more stimulating effect. In all your healing sessions, continue to visualize the energy coming from your palms and fingertips. It's important to become accustomed to the hand movements so that you can then shift your focus to the visualization of this energy pouring from the hands.

Exercise #2: Short strokes similar to the longer ones described in the previous exercise can be used to energize or cleanse smaller areas of the body or small organs.

To do this, you simply place your focus on the part of the body you want to treat. Make short gentle strokes in the air above the area with the palms outward and the fingers gently spread. Visualize rays of light energy flowing out of your fingertips.

This motion differs from the long stroke in that when you raise your hand in these short strokes, you can raise it with your palm turned slightly toward you. The idea is to avoid energizing the area with an upward motion because this can cause congestion.

After a few short strokes, fling your fingers to the side as if you are flicking off water to get rid of excess or depleted energy.

Do these motions until you are comfortable. Once you are accustomed to them and they feel natural to you, add the visualization of the beam of energetic light, tinged with a hint of blue.

You may find difficulty coordinating these activities of moving the hands and visualizing, at first, but after a little practice, it becomes easier. The most important thing is to be able to see the energy flowing out of your hands. This visualization becomes stronger with practice, until the image is densely impressed on your mind and the coordination of the hand movements with the emanation of this energy becomes automatic.

Exercise #3: A body that is depleted of energy, tired and fatigued can be re-energized, stimulated and strengthened by directing energy at the thyroid gland, which is the master gland of the system and controls metabolism.

Re-energize the thyroid gland by placing your right

palm outward facing the organ, which rests behind the skin, muscle and bone at the throat, right where a person would wear a bow-tie.

See this organ in your mind's eye and project a beam of light three to four inches in diameter directly at the organ. There is no need to move your hand, only visualize this beam of light tinged with a slight blue flowing out of the palm.

As you do this, visualize a ball of light over your head, which allows energy to flow through your head and through your entire body. You can, also, see energy flowing through your left hand and feel it coming into your body through the soles of your feet.

It is important to perform this exercise along with these visualizations because if you energize other people with only the energy from your own body, you will soon become weak and energetically depleted. Methods of increasing your supply of vital energy will be discussed in the following chapters. For now, maintain this visualization of energy flowing into your body through your head, left hand and your feet as best you can.

This is a good exercise for helping you to coordinate these visualizations: The flow of energy into your body and the directed flow of it outward into the depleted organ.

It may take one to two minutes or as long as 15 minutes to re-energize the thyroid by this method depending on how depleted the organ is. You can determine this through visualization, by holding your palm an inch or two away from the gland and feeling its energy level or you can energize the organ until you feel that it begins to resist you. This is something like filling a tank with gas. You can sense when the tank is nearly full. Stop when you feel that the gland is unable to accept anymore energy.

In a similar fashion, you can stimulate small or

delicate organs using your fingertips. The procedure is the same as above, except you point one or two fingers at the organ and see the beam of light extending from them into the organ.

A more powerful variation on this is to raise your hand in a similar fashion as described before, with all five fingers delicately pointing toward the area of the body to be affected (almost as if you are softly holding a ball in your palm), then force beams of energy from your fingers in a twisting motion into the body as if you were boring holes.

Exercise #4: Remove depleted and diseased energy from cells, organs, tissues and chakras. It is advisable to cleanse an organ or chakra before re-energizing it. This technique removes dirty, diseased energy and makes more room for healthy vital force.

Sometimes just this one act of removing unhealthy energies from organs that are engorged with too much energy provides relief. This technique can, also, be used to remove blockages in the system.

To do this, first raise your right palm so that it faces outward toward the organ or chakra to be cleansed, then lower your index and middle finger so that it points directly at the area you wish to affect. Then rotate your hand in a counter-clockwise motion. Circle from your wrist as you direct your two fingers.

This time, visualize energy flowing out of the organ and toward your hand. Make 20 or more such circles, seeing the depleted energy being pulled out of the organ in a stream. Allow it to accumulate into a little cloudy ball in the palm of your hand. Then, shake it off, again, as if you were flicking water from your fingers. After you release it, visualize the ball of depleted energy going up into a little "poof" of flames.

Resume making little counter-clockwise circles and

continue to pull the energy out. Again, after 20 or more circular motions, throw the ball of energy away from you and visually destroy it.

Continue doing this until you sense it is time to stop.

As you are doing this exercise, you do not need to visualize energy coming into your body as you do when you are energizing someone.

Take caution not to pull energy out too quickly. Doing so can cause unpleasant sensations, nausea and even pain in your subject. Listen to your own body, your own senses and to what other people tell you when you perform these techniques.

Exercise #5: This is a powerful way to energize the chakras and any part of the body. It involves doing the opposite of what you did in the previous exercise. But, since you are energizing, you will need to visualize a supply of vital energy flowing into your own body from your head, left hand and feet.

To do this, first raise your right palm so that it faces outward toward the organ or chakra to be energized, then lower your index and middle finger so that it points directly at the area you wish to affect. Then rotate your hand in a clockwise motion. Circle from your wrist as you direct your two fingers.

This time, visualize energy flowing out of your palms and fingers and into the organ as you rotate your hand from the wrist in a clockwise direction. This light is white, but tinged with a slight blue hue. You may make hundreds of circles at the body, all the while visualizing yourself as a channel for the vital force. The blue tinged light flows into your left hand and out your right. It flows into the top of your head and in through the bottoms of your feet and out of the palms and fingers of your right hand.

Close your eyes and see this action taking place.

Visualize yourself doing this healing and see it during your leisure time when you are at rest. Soon, you will be able to hold this visualization with your eyes open as you are doing this healing.

When you are cleansing and energizing an organ, you may alternate *Exercise #4* with this exercise, thus removing unhealthy, depleted energy and replacing it with fresh, vibrant Life Force energy. End the cycle when the organ or chakra is energized and functioning properly.

Other Movements:

Another way to energize the body is to vigorously rub the hands together to activate the energy centers in the palms of your hands, then place them a few inches away from the part of the body you want to influence. Allow the life energy to simply radiate out of the palms of your hands and saturate the depleted area.

As you move your hands in the previously described exercises, you will begin to acquire your own style. One movement that may develop as you learn to focus your concentration on the energy you are imparting or extracting is a quick fluttering or vibrating movement of the hand. Also, as you are pulling energy out, you may find yourself making quick motions as if to say, "Come here." These are more advanced movements that are acquired by practice. Allow them to develop naturally.

5

HOW TO INCREASE YOUR VITAL
FORCE

It is important for both your physical strength and
success at magical healing to possess a substantial
supply of the vital force. A powerful supply may be
accumulated by means of your directed will through
visualization coupled with controlled breathing.

Practice the following meditation of rhythmic
breathing to increase your personal supply of vital
energy:

Breathing Meditation

Sit or stand in a relaxed but erect position with your
chest, neck and head in alignment and your shoulders
slightly thrown back. Let your hands rest naturally and
easily on your upper thighs or lap. Do not slouch.

Practice breathing deeply through your nose. Deep
breathing is something almost no one in the modern,

civilized world does naturally, so it may feel a little uncomfortable at first, as your muscles and organs get accustomed to taking in more air.

Inhale slowly and deeply, first filling the upper chamber of the lungs, then the lower chamber and finally the stomach. (We are usually taught to use our muscles to pull the stomach in, but for the duration of this meditation, you should forget that old instruction and allow your stomach to fill with air.) Then, release the breath through your mouth in the reverse order: Exhale slowly from the stomach, then the lower part of the lungs, then the upper part of the lungs.

After you feel comfortable breathing deeply this way and it has become more natural for you, proceed to add the element of rhythm to your breathing.

Adding Rhythm:

To find your body's personal rhythm, feel or listen for your own pulse while you are in this relaxed state. Establish that rhythm in your mind as you count out the beats: 1, 2, 3, 4, 5, 6.

Now, take a deep breath as before, but this time mete your inhalation in time to the rhythm of your pulse to the count of six. Count "1" as you inhale and stop inhaling when you reach "6."

Hold this breath for the count of "3."

Then, release your breath, just as before, only this time rhythmically counting. As you begin to exhale, count "1" and when you have no more air in your lungs you should be at "6."

Then, hold your lungs empty for the count of "3" before beginning all over, again.

You will probably not be able to coordinate your rhythmic counting with your inhaling and exhaling perfectly the first few times you do this. You may not have it right for the first 100 times, either. But, that is fine. It doesn't have to be perfect to be effective and you will become more proficient as you do it.

Don't overdo this exercise in the beginning. Depending on what kind of physical condition you are in, you may want to start with only three repetitions. Try to work up to doing 15 at a session after a week or two, but do not force your body if it becomes fatigued. If you begin to feel dizzy, stop immediately and resume normal breathing.

This exercise alone helps to increase your body's strength and vitality. But, it is increased even more so when it is coupled with visualization.

Adding Visualization:

As you breathe, close your eyes and form such a clear mental image of the flow of energy into your body that you can actually feel a warm, tingling sensation. You may choose to see it coming in through the top of your head, through the soles of your feet, through your hands or through any other chakra center, organ or part of your body that is especially in need of revitalization.

Visualize it as a blue-tinged beam of light. It may be similar to the translucent beam of light that shines through trees illuminated by the sun. Or, it might appear more substantial, like the light emitted from a laser. You may, also, visualize it as a billowing cloud.

As you exhale, see some of this energy going out of the same part of the body. In this way, you are cleansing your body's energy in that location by the force of your breath.

As an exercise, lie comfortably on your back, close your eyes and inhale. Now, visualize light, like the rays of the sun, warming your body. First, feel it in your left foot. Allow your foot to become very warm and energized. Then move the energy to your right foot. Let your foot really absorb this energy until it feels warm just as if it were exposed to the light of the sun.

Then, move the light to your left hand and allow yourself to feel the same sensations there. Then, move it to your right hand, to your left shoulder and finally to your right shoulder.

Now, return to your rhythmic breathing, again. This time mentally direct the flow of energy into your body. You may choose any part of your body you like. If you don't know where to start, begin visualizing a flow of energy in through the palm of your left hand and out through your right.

The following is an example of how to mentally direct the flow of energy:

Inhale upon the count of "1." See and feel a wide beam of blue light entering your left palm. It has a strong electro-static energy that pulses up your arm and to your elbow.

Count "2." More energy flows continually into your left palm, up to your elbow and into your left shoulder.

Count "3." The energy fills your chest, you can feel the vibrant electrical pulsations.

Count "4." The energy continues to fill your entire body from your head to your toes.

Count "5." The energy moves into your right shoulder.

Count "6." It moves down your right arm and into your right hand.

Hold this breath for the count of "3."

Then, exhale and as you do, see a flow of energy proceeding out of your right arm from the elbow and out through the palm and fingers of your right hand. Count rhythmically from 1 to 6, seeing and feeling this energy as it moves out of your hand, flowing constantly until you reach the count of 6.

Hold this position for the count of "3" as the flow of energy out of your hand ceases.

Then, begin again, just as before. Inhale upon the count of "1," feeling and seeing the electrifying sensation of energy flowing into your left hand.

Continue this exercise for, at least, three repetitions before taking a break. You ultimate goal is to be able to do, at least, 15 repetitions uninterrupted.

Do not be frustrated if your mind wanders. Simply, put it right back on track with your breathing, counting and visualizing. Eventually, you will be able to do this without any disruptive thoughts and without fatigue. Always stop if you begin to feel dizzy.

Exercise to Improve Your Visualization

Your visualizations will become more vivid with practice. It is all a matter of memory recall. This short exercise is intended to help you improve your ability to visualize colors.

1. Begin by closing your eyes, then:

2. Visualize an apple. Then, visualize the color red.

3. Visualize an orange. Then, visualize the color orange.

4. Visualize a banana. Then, visualize the color yellow.

5. Visualize a tree. Then, visualize the color green.

6. Visualize the sky. Then, visualize the color blue.

7. Visualize a plum. Then, visualize the color purple.

8. Visualize a violet. Then, visualize the color violet.

9. Visualize a white wedding gown. Then, visualize the color white.

If you can visualize any of the above, you can visualize anything. Believe you can do it and you can.

Breathing Exercise for Increased Energy and Wisdom

Sit in a comfortable recliner or lie upon your bed. Breathe rhythmically and meditate on what is called your "higher self" or your soul. For the moment, think of your body as a vehicle, which you as a spirit, your higher self, inhabit and which you can leave and return to whenever you choose.

Continue breathing. Feel yourself only as a spirit, light and airy. You will soon become almost unaware of your body. Feel your spirit rise lightly in the air. Enjoy this feeling knowing that when you are ready, you can descend back into your body.

With each breath you inhale, visualize universal strength and power entering your body, borne by the vital force. As you exhale imagine yourself imparting that force filled with love for every living thing. Let the power of the universe circulate around and permeate every part of you.

Enjoy this sensation for a few minutes.

Then, place your mind in a state of reverence to the creative forces of the universe. Open yourself to the influx of divine wisdom. Let the knowledge and wisdom of the universe pour into your soul, your mind and your body from above in shimmering, dazzling rays of light.

As you meditate, allow your mind to dwell upon

these ideas until they become manifest and gradually clearer in your mind's eye. Soon, your mind will be passive and at rest. And, as you continue to practice these meditations at intervals of once or twice per week, you will find it easier and easier to enter the meditative state, to leave your body and to receive the outpouring of wisdom and love from the universe.

OTHER METHODS OF MANIPULATING THE VITAL FORCE

Once you have mastered the previous methods of healing through the projection of the vital force and have amassed your own powerful supply of vital energy, you can begin exploring other methods of magical healing.

As you practice, you will find it increasingly easier to coordinate your activities and your ability to focus your mind and direct energy will become greater.

Commanding Intelligences

As previously mentioned, cells and organs have a kind of intelligence or mind with which the healer can communicate.

A few books have been written about how some diseases are specifically related to beliefs, emotions or subconsciously held ideas. There may be some element of truth in this notion.

It is somewhat true that "thoughts are things," at least, thought-forms, which are masses of subtle energy directed by the mind, are truly things. If people sometimes inadvertently create their illnesses by means of thought-forms, then it stands to reason that such illnesses may be un-created the same way.

Each cell, organ, nerve center, ganglia, kind of tissue, etc., has its own intelligence and can respond to a strongly directed command carried along by a powerful force of vital energy. In this manner, you may direct your energized commands at your own cells and organs or someone else's in order to achieve magical healing.

When it is done correctly, healing can take place very quickly. Your purpose is to re-establish the proper mental attitude of the cells or the organ, itself. This is not a question of mind over matter. It is an assertion of your will directed upon the living intelligence of those cells or that organ.

When you are healing yourself by this method, you are not doing so by changing your own thoughts or emotional patterns; and, when you are healing someone else, you are not altering their thoughts or emotions. You are only affecting the energetic mind of the misbehaving cells or organ. It is there you must direct your will.

Let's say for purposes of illustration that you want to restore a malfunctioning gall bladder. You would direct your thoughts upon the gall bladder in order to establish mental resonance. Hold the idea of it in your mind for a moment. Then, speak the words aloud or use your inner voice to command the gall bladder to work properly.

Address the gall bladder as if you were trying to get its attention, "Gall bladder, you are causing trouble and you must begin acting correctly. You must start doing your job properly, at once. You are to keep this body in good working order. Do your job right!"

You may speak to the organ sharply or gently, but

you should speak to it lovingly. After all, what you are telling it is for its own good. So, you should take that attitude and never speak angrily to cells or an organ.

Another gentler method is to give cells and organs permission to heal. Tell them that they have suffered long enough and it is time for them to restore themselves to their normal, youthful, vibrant state. This method works especially well on the heart, which is prone to illness due to emotional or mental suffering.

Again, with this type of treatment, you must address the mind of the cells and organs and not the mind of the person.

The Practice of Mesmerism

Mesmerism is the coupling of hypnotic suggestion with the manipulation of the vital force, which Mesmer called "magnetic fluid." Hypnosis is a natural, relaxed state, which can be reached through suggestion as well as other methods.

Once a person is in even a slight hypnotic trance, healing suggestions can be made, which are very powerful when coupled with the manipulation of the vital force. Although, it is not always discussed, some hypnotists use a combination of these things in their hypnosis practices. Another term for the practice of thought transference of this kind is "telepathy."

The hypnotic state allows the healer to manipulate the subconscious mind. Begin by sweeping your subject as you did in *Chapter 4, Exercise #1*. Make suggestions that correspond with your intentions. For example, while you are performing these movements and the accompanying visualization, in a soothing voice, tell your subject that he is becoming more relaxed. This time, you are communicating with the person's mind; not necessarily the cells or organs of the body as described in the previous chapter.

If you are dealing with a subject who has come to you in a frazzled, frantic state, say, "I am going to help you. In a matter of minutes you will feel better."

Ask for your subject's full attention as you proceed. As you are stroking the energies around the person, say, "You are calm, relaxed and completely at peace." Use a hypnotic voice that is a little bit quieter and lower than your normal voice. Draw out the sounds a little longer than you normally would. Your speech should be rhythmic, but it should have a natural emotional quality to it.

Imagine yourself treating a patient:

When you perform your treatments, find a place that is quiet and free from the intrusive sounds of strange voices, barking dogs, traffic and other disruptive noises. If possible, dim the lights and pull down the shades.

Imagine that you are standing and he is sitting in a chair in front of you.

See yourself performing the stroking motions of *Chapter 4, Exercise #1.* See the energy flowing into your body and out your right hand.

Now, tell your subject in your best hypnotic voice that the result he desires will be accomplished. Repeat these words several times in different ways. Speak gently, but punctuate the words with emotion so that he can feel what you are saying. For example, "Your health is being fully restored. Now, you are feeling strong and vibrant."

In giving the suggestions, keep in mind the desired outcome. With your words, combined with your manipulation of the life force, lead your subject by degrees to this condition. As you do so, picture in your own mind the desired outcome. Your thoughts become manifest in your actions and your subject follows the imagined progress in his own mind.

There is a constant transmission of the force of thoughts associated with your words occurring as you do this. But, the effect is being enhanced by the powerfully suggestive words you are using as you mentally manipulate the life force.

Under the power of suggestion, the subject's mind is also working to enhance this energetic manipulation and more quickly achieve the desired outcome. The subject's mind becomes an agent in his own healing process.

It is important when you are making suggestions to a person under hypnosis not to make reference to the diseased condition or speak in the negative. These positive mental suggestions are called "affirmations." Affirmations should only affirm positive conditions; never negative ones.

For instance, you should not say, "You no longer feel pain." This is because the subconscious will understand this as an order to "feel pain." Instead say, "You feel perfectly comfortable and at ease."

Always endeavor to lead the subject's mind away from the undesired condition and allow it to focus only on the desired outcome.

Incorrect Affirmation: "You are not weak."

Correct Affirmation: "You are strong."

Example of a Mesmeric Treatment

The following is a example of how to treat someone using a combination of vital energy manipulation and mental suggestion. It is not necessary to use a script. Adapt your words to each individual's needs. Remember to only use words that will help them to be calm and relaxed and avoid using any words or subject that might cause discomfort or antagonism.

After you have quieted your subject and you are going the calming, stroking motions with your hands that are used to calm and relax a person, say: "Now, _____, you are resting quietly and easily. Your entire body is at rest. Every muscle is relaxed. Every nerve is quiet. You are feeling entirely relaxed and restful from your head to your toes... you feel quiet, restful and easy. Your mind is calm and composed and you will allow the words I say to sink deep, deep down into your subconscious mind so they may bring about a state of strength and total health."

Now, begin treating your subject's navel chakra. Use the counter-clockwise motion from *Chapter 4, Exercise #4* to remove any dirty or depleted energy. As you do so, say: "I will begin by strengthening your digestion. Your stomach is going to become stronger and stronger, imparting strength and vigor to every cell and fiber of your body. From now on your stomach will digest the proper amount of food that your body needs. It will properly assimilate the nutrients and convert it to nourishment and energy for the vigor and vitality of your entire body."

Now, re-energize the navel chakra using the clockwise motion from *Chapter 4, Exercise #5* and as you do so, say: "Your stomach is stronger and stronger now. It is willing and able to do its best work for you. It digests your food perfectly and provides optimum nutrition and strength to every cell of your body. You can feel its increasing strength and power as it becomes stronger and stronger so that it does its job better and better each day. Your stomach is sending nourishment to all parts of your body and impulses to any tired cells or organs giving them renewed strength, health and power."

You can move on and treat any other parts of the

body or the chakra system that require treatment. When you are finished, leave your subject with a healing suggestion while you perform a final sweeping, as you did in *Chapter 4, Exercise #1*. Say: "You are stronger all over, from head to foot and every organ, cell and part is functioning properly now. Health, strength, energy and vigor are flowing into your body right now and they will continue to do so. Your body will continue to heal, rejuvenate and strengthen itself."

You now have the key to healing as Mesmer did and you can adapt it to virtually any treatment your subjects need. Experience will lead you intuitively to the right suggestions to make and the best way to go about it. No two healers do things exactly the same way.

The Eyes as a Mechanism for Energy and Thought Transference

Mesmer was known for his ability to fascinate or fixate his subjects. When he made suggestions he held their attention with his gaze because he understood that the eyes were capable of transmitting the "magnetic force."

You can use your eyes as Mesmer did when you give suggestions. Cultivate a firm earnest gaze, but do not stare. The difference is that a gaze is active, engaged and attentive, whereas a stare is an inactive, absent-minded state. Practice looking at people's eyes in an interested, attentive way.

The eyes can be used to transmit helpful or harmful energies. The latter idea is the basis for belief in the "Evil Eye" in many cultures around the world.

Treatment by the eye is used by some healers, almost exactly as the hands are used. It is both a means of transmission of the vital force and a method of unwaveringly focusing the will.

The healer sweeps the subject with his or her gaze. By the same method, an analysis of areas of the body that are diseased, imbalanced or depleted of energy can be made. The part of the body that needs healing is then energized by the fixed gaze of the healer upon that part. It is bathed in rays of healing energy emitted from the healer's eyes.

The Healing Breath

The breath is another means of transmitting the vital force.

Place a clean towel or napkin over the part of the body to be healed. Then, press your half-parted lips on the towel and slowly blow healing energy into it as if you are penetrating the body with it. Your breath will suffuse the towel, which will become very warm.

Another method doesn't require a towel. You simply blow upon the area requiring treatment. This can be done at a distance of one or two inches or a few feet.

This method is used to clear congestion and drive out impure energies.

Magnetizing Organs

Organs of the body, particularly those of the pelvis, including the bladder, bowel, intestines and uterus can sometimes become dislodged from their proper place, "prolapsed" or "dropped." A healer can magnetize these organs with her hands and draw them upward.

The person to be healed should lie on her back. Place your palms facing downward over the area to be healed. Hold them at a distance of anywhere from 6 inches to a foot away. Now, focus your mind on the organs to be moved. Let your mind resonate with them. Then move your hands in a pulling motion in short upward strokes as if you are coaxing the organ to move.

If you mentally resonate with the organs, you can move them in a matter of seconds. The subject will feel it. There should be no pain associated with this movement and if your subject is in pain, it should soon be relieved.

When the organs have moved, energize the area by holding your hands steadily over it and silently willing the organs to stay in their proper place.

Increasing and Decreasing the Flow of Blood

Using the body's magnetism to increase or decrease the blood flow, thin or thicken the blood. Just as all of the spinning particles that comprise the atoms of your body on the physical and metaphysical levels have polarity similar to that of a battery, so does your body as a whole.

For this reason, you are able to use the polarity in your body to increase or decrease the blood flow in another person by following these instructions:

In any case, the person to be healed should be placed on his or her back. The knees should be brought up so the spine is straight.

Blood Thickening:

This might be used in the case of an emergency where a person is bleeding and it must be slowed or stopped. To thicken the blood of a person, place yourself on his right side. Then, place your left hand with the palm facing downward at the top of the head. Place your right hand with the palm facing upward at the base of the spine. There is no need to physically touch the person. Hold this position for five minutes or until the desired result is obtained.

Blood Thinning:

To thin the blood, do the opposite. Go to the person's left side. Then, place your right hand with the palm facing downward at the top of the head. Place your left hand with the palm facing upward at the base of the spine. There is no need to physically touch the person. Hold this position for five minutes or until the desired result is obtained.

MAGICAL TOOLS

Pendulums and other divination tools are used to dowse for information about health conditions. The formal term for this kind of diagnosis is "medical radiesthesia." The term was coined in 1927 by a French priest, the Abbe Alex Bouly who together with the Abbe Alexis Mermet pioneered its practice.

The term radiesthesia means "to perceive radiation" and it pertains to other forms of dowsing. It is often used in reference to medical dowsing, but it is sometimes used to refer to dowsing, in general.

The hypothesis of medical radiesthesia is: All things emit radiation; a current of energy flows through human hands; and objects can become tools by which to obtain information about a subject.

We have already mentioned one form of medical radiesthesia in which you hold your hands, palms facing a person, and feel for the strength of their auric field. The other form involves the use of an instrument such as a pendulum.

Basics of Using a Pendulum

It is best to acquire a pendulum that is properly weighted and balanced, but almost anything can be used as a pendulum. It is simply a weight suspended from a length of string or chain. You "tune" the pendulum by adjusting its length. A shorter length swings faster than a longer one. This is a matter of personal preference.

The pendulum appears to work on the basis of energy and impulses sent through the body as a result of directed thought.

Whenever you use a pendulum, you must formulate a question and then wait, with the attitude of an observer, for the response.

A pendulum does not work exactly the same way for every person. There are two ways to determine pendulum indications for you:

The first is to simply ask the pendulum. Hold the pendulum suspended in front of you and command it. Say, "Show me what 'Yes' is for me." Then wait and watch what the pendulum does. It may go in a clockwise or counter-clockwise circle, it may swing back and forth or it may remain still. This is your "Yes" indication.

Then command it to show you your "No" response. Say, "Show me what 'No' is for me." Then, wait and watch what the pendulum does. Again, it may go in a clockwise or counter-clockwise circle, it may swing back and forth or it may remain still. This is your "No" indication.

The second method is to program the pendulum to move as you want it to for certain indications. Commonly used indications are to have the pendulum swing back and forth for "Yes," from side to side for "No" and around in a circle when the question cannot be answered.

In medical radiesthesia, it is common to have the pendulum swing back and forth when it is "neutral," in a clockwise direction for "Yes" and in a counter-clockwise direction for "No."

Make these pendulum motions intentionally, at first. Practice like this for a few minutes.

Pause and then, with a serious mind, test your pendulum by asking it a question you already know the answer to. For example, "Is my name _____?" Then, wait for the answer.

Hold the pendulum over a common object like a book and ask, "Is this a book?" Wait for the answer. Then, hold the pendulum over the same object and as, "Is this a rock?"

After you do this several times and receive consistently correct responses from the pendulum, it is programmed.

Performing Medical Radiesthesia

Use the pendulum to diagnose the condition of chakras, organs and systems of the body or to determine which remedies to give or other steps to take.

Pendulum Diagnosis Exercise #1:

Ask your willing test subject to recline on a sofa. If you do not have another person to help you, then you should recline on the sofa. Take the pendulum in your right hand.

You are going to determine how well each chakra center is functioning. An over or under-functioning chakra, eventually leads to disease in the organs associated with it.

The order is not important, but for purpose of this exercise, let's begin at the base Chakra, which is located at the bottom of the spine. Hold the pendulum over it and ask to be shown the motion of the chakra. The pendulum should begin spinning in a clockwise direction very rapidly.

If a chakra is only malfunctioning slightly, it may be spinning slowly or it may even be spinning backwards (counter-clockwise).

After you have received your response, then move to the next, the sacral chakra, which is a little above the previous one and is associated with the sex organs. Ask to be shown the motion of this chakra.

Then, move to every other one in succession, doing the same thing with the pendulum. Ask to be shown the motion of the energy centers of the navel, spleen, solar plexus, the heart, the throat, the third eye and, finally the crown, which is situated above the top of the head.

Once you have determined the direction and speed of the motion of each, you have performed your first pendulum diagnosis.

Any chakra that is not turning rapidly in a clockwise motion is said to be out of balance. When one is out of balance usually others are malfunctioning trying to account for the over-functioning or under-functioning of its brother.

The following shows how the pendulum can be used to heal:

Take your pendulum in hand, once again, and place it over any chakra that is not functioning properly. Allow the pendulum to show you the movement of the chakra, again. When it does this, you know you have the image of the chakra fixed in your mind and you have found resonance with it. Now, you can manipulate its energy with the pendulum by forcing it to rotate faster and in the right direction. Force this motion for a minute. Then, take a receptive mental attitude with the pendulum once again and ask it to show you its movement. It should be spinning properly now.

Do the same with each malfunctioning chakra to bring them all into balance.

Pendulum Diagnosis Exercise #2:

Place your left hand into the right palm of the person you want to test. You can also test yourself by placing your left hand on yourself. Or, use a photograph of the person you want to test, a recent full-body shot is best.

Then, hold your pendulum over the name of each Vitamin or Mineral below and ask, "Does the person need more of this?"

(This is by no means a complete list and is only presented as an exercise.)

Vitamins:

Vitamin A
Vitamin B1 (Thiamin)
Vitamin B6
Vitamin B12 (Cobalamin)
Vitamin C
Vitamin D
Vitamin E
Folic Acid (Folacin)
Vitamin K
Biotin
Niacin
Pantothenic Acid
Riboflavin

Minerals:

Boron
Calcium
Chloride
Iodine
Magnesium
Phosphorous
Potassium
Sodium

Alternatively, you may hold the bottle of a nutritional supplement in your hand and test it on yourself or another person by asking the pendulum.

In any case, for your radiesthesia to be effective you must make a mental connection between the person to be analyzed and the substance you are testing.

The application of the pendulum to gain information is a very simple one and you can devise all kinds of systems of your own for determining answers based on the binary response of "Yes" or "No." There are spiral-bound books that are nothing but pendulum charts for various purposes, but you can easily draw up your own. Alternatively, people use the letters from the Scrabble board or a Ouija board to ask more complex questions.

Dowsing with the pendulum, rods, twigs and a singular device, called a bobber, has long been employed to find water, minerals, hidden treasure, lost objects and missing people. Dowsing is a very natural thing to do, but the ability has been lost or blocked by many people because of the prevalence of superstitious religious beliefs. You should be able to pick this ability up in a matter of minutes, but if you would like to learn more about it, the American Society of Dowsers is a nationwide organization that teaches people how to dowse. (www.dowsers.org) A similar organization exists in the U.K. (www.britishdowsers.org)

Healing Wands

The purpose of a healing wand is to direct and magnify vital force energy. Using a wand can take some of the work out of healing because, when it is properly designed, it does a lot of the work of directing and projecting energy for you.

Two basic types of wands work well for this purpose. Both use quartz crystals in their construction, but one relies more on the power of the stones and the other involves the use of a combination of organic and inorganic materials to accumulate orgone energy.

The first type, quartz crystal healing wands, are usually comprised of an elongated, shaped gemstone. Commonly used stones are amethyst, jasper, agate, blood stone and rose quartz but others are used, too. Typically, it is wrapped with silver or copper, decorated with smaller colored gemstones and terminates at one end with a single clear quartz, from which the energy is projected at the target. These wands are available at metaphysical stores, including online stores like AzureGreen.com and are commonly sold as "Chakra Wands." But, their use is not limited to the manipulation of chakras.

The other type of wand, which is more economical and sometimes more powerful, involves the construction of orgonite. Orgonite is an energy accumulator. The energy is gathered and cleansed in a matrix of organic and inorganic materials.

Organic materials are carbon-based substances. Clay and resin are the most commonly used in orgonite construction.

Non-organic substances are metals. Copper, steel and aluminum are commonly used in orgonite devices.

Instructions for Making a Powerful Orgonite Crystal Wand

To construct your orgone wand, you will need the following:

1. Bakeable clay, for example, Sculpey brand (available at craft and hobby stores)

2. A piece of copper tubing about 1/2" in diameter and 6 to 8 inches long

3. A piece of copper hobby wire 16 to 20 inches long (available at craft and hobby stores)

4. Copper bee-bees or metal filings (steel, copper or aluminum)

5. Crushed or very small pieces of quartz gemstones. This is an ideal use for small broken pieces. They should be small enough to fit into the copper tube

6. A gemstone to serve as the "cap" of the wand. You may use a small crystal ball or a tumbled gemstone

7. A single-terminated, clear quartz crystal that is wide enough to fit on the end of your copper tube and is about an inch or more in length

8. Adhesive such as epoxy that is used to glue metal to gemstones (available at craft and hobby stores)

9. A conventional stove in which to heat the clay once you have molded it

10. A pair of wire clippers

11. A pair of needle-nosed pliers used in wire-jewelry making

When you are choosing materials for your wand, keep in mind that larger pieces of crystal seem to have more power. Larger wands are usually more powerful than smaller ones. Let your intuition guide you in the selection of these items.

Begin by taking your needle nosed pliers and forming a coil with your hobby wire. To do this, grasp the end of the wire with your pliers and begin turning it end over end until you have made a little coil. It doesn't have to be perfect.

Pull the coil upward approximately the length of the tube.

Glue one end of this coil to the "cap" stone and wait for it to dry.

Place the tube over the wire that is attached to the stone, so that the stone now sits at the bottom of the tube forming the "cap" at the base of your wand. The coiled wire should be slightly protruding from the other end of the tube. Place some adhesive on the "cap" stone and the bottom of the copper tube and allow it to dry.

Fill your wand with more or less equal sprinklings of a combination of the metal filings and tiny gemstone pieces. You can drizzle a little glue inside to keep them from moving around. Try to keep the wire in the middle. Leave a little room (approximately 1/4") at the top.

Using your pliers, slightly coil the end of the wire that is sticking out of the tube. If it is too long, clip it. Then, glue your large quartz crystal, with its point facing outward, onto the end of the both the coil and the tube. Allow this to dry.

Finish by covering the copper tube in clay. To do this, roll the clay out flat as if you were rolling out pie dough, then shape it a round the tube. Leave the cap stone at the bottom and the large quartz crystal at the top exposed.

You may decorate the clay with more gemstones or pewter charms.

Then, bake the wand on a rack in your oven according to the instructions on your package of clay. Sculpey clay bakes in about 20 to 30 minutes depending on its thickness.

When it is cool, test your newly constructed wand as you would any other.

How to Test the Strength of a Wand

When selecting a healing wand, test it to judge its strength. One way to test a wand's strength is to point it straight at your thymus gland. Hold the point a distance of about 6 inches away. You might feel pressure and, if you have any congestion in your lungs, you might begin to cough almost immediately as the energy from the wand clears it out. If this happens in a matter of seconds, this is a sign of a powerful wand.

Another way to test it is by holding the wand in your right hand and pointing it at the palm of your left hand. A powerful wand will give you a strong sense of heat, a prickly or electrical sensation.

Test the beam of the wand visually by holding it against a white background. A strong wand produces a broad, blue, laser-like beam from the end of the crystal.

You can also test its strength on a scale of 1 to 10 using your pendulum. Hold the pendulum over the wand and say, "Show me the strength of this wand on a scale of 1 to 10 where 10 is the greatest." Then proceed to ask, "Is it 1, 2, 3...?" until you get a positive response.

How to Use a Wand

Use your wand just as you would use your hands in magical healing. You may use the wand to make cleansing and energizing motions exactly as you were shown in previous exercises. Circle to the left to cleanse an organ, cell or chakra. Do the opposite to energize it.

Alternatively, you may use the wand passively to draw energy out of an area by holding the base a few inches away from it with the point outward. The wand will do its job without your aide, however, you may assist by visualizing the wand drawing the diseased energy out of the body.

Powerfully charge the master gland by aiming the wand at your thymus for 3 to 15 minutes. The body immediately feels more energized.

Charge any part of the body the same way, by steadily holding the pointed end of the wand a few inches away from it and directing energy at it for a few minutes.

Again, you may assist by visualizing healing energy being formulated within the wand and coming out through the crystal in a blue beam. But, this is not absolutely necessary because your wand generates and emits energy at all times.

Because it is a passive instrument, you can energize your own chakras and organs by simply aiming the wand at those areas. Do this while you're conducting your breathing exercises (six breaths in, rest for three, six breaths out, rest for three, etc.) or while you are relaxed and watching television or reading a book.

Use your pendulum to determine when these areas are sufficiently energized or cleansed.

Crystal Balls

Another way to increase your personal power, either while you are meditating, resting passively or conducting a healing session, is by holding a crystal ball.

There are two types of quartz crystal balls available: Natural and reconstituted.

Natural crystals are those that have been shaped from a whole piece of quartz and have natural imperfections. They may be clear quartz crystal or any other type of semi-precious gemstone. Like wands, their power is usually relative to their size. But, some crystals seem to be more energetic than others.

Reconstituted clear quartz crystal balls are very nearly perfect looking. Most very large crystal balls you see are made of reconstituted quartz. Interestingly, reconstituted quartz is often more lively and energetic than natural quartz.

The strength of crystal balls is something you must test yourself, either by placing your hands on or over the crystal balls and comparing them or by the use of your pendulum.

Cleanse any crystal with your breath and your intention in a matter of seconds. Blow on the crystal as you imagine the old energy moving out of it swiftly in the shape of a cloud.

Alternatively, cleanse a crystal as you would cleanse a part of the body. Simply, wave your hand over it a few times making short passes away from you. Envision the old programming clearing. Then hold your right hand over the crystal (or place both hands on a larger one, if you prefer) and command the crystal to increase its power.

This can be done with any smaller crystals, gemstones, your wand or your pendulum. Simply command it to have more energy. Place items you want to energize near the crystal to passively increase their vital force.

Meditate or sleep near natural, "feminine" crystal balls to help keep your personal life force energy charged. Feminine crystals are the heavily clouded crystals as opposed to the masculine ones which are clearer. Feminine quartz is powerful, but it emanates its energetic charge more slowly, so it should not disturb your ability to sleep.

Charge up your crystal ball's energy by placing a large piece of selenite or apophyllite near it. A large selenite wand placed from head to toe underneath your bed will, also, charge and balance your chakras while you sleep.

Magnetizing Objects and Distance Healing

An object like a pendant, ring, handkerchief or scarf can be magnetized or energized by a healer and then given to a person to wear. The object will diffuse the healing energy placed in it by the healer to the wearer.

Similarly, a person can easily be treated at a distance, if you can obtain a photograph, signature, intimate personal item, nail clippings, hair or saliva or a few drops of blood on a clean cotton ball. Diagnose and treat these items just as you would treat the person. Such items become what is know as a "witness" or a substitute for the person.

Some healers create a poppet or a doll with these items, affixing a photograph and inserting personal items belonging to the person to be healed into the doll. Then, the doll is treated just as if the patient it represents were in front of you.

Treatments may be successfully performed at a distance by advanced magical healers who can very closely envision the person to be treated. The technique is very similar to healing yourself through astral projection, which is discussed it *Chapter 8*. In this instance, you locate the astral body of your patient through time and space and mentally heal him using the same techniques you would use to heal yourself. It takes a little practice, but it is highly effective. Pain, rashes, fatigue and a wide variety of adverse conditions are relieved in a matter of seconds when it is done by an adept.

Stones and Colors in Healing

The study of gemstones and their role in healing is a vast one. If you want to go into great depth on this subject the books by the author, Melody, are unsurpassed. Most of them are academic, but one of them, called *Love is in the Earth*, is about the healing properties of gemstones.

St. Albertus Magnus' book, *Secrets of the Virtues of Herbs, Stones and Certain Beasts*, was first published in London, England in 1604. Aristotle and Pliny wrote about the healing powers of crystals and this knowledge is surely far more ancient.

Working with gemstones for healing is so natural, you will soon find that your ability to succeed with them is instinctual.

All but clear quartz crystals come in a wide variety of colors. The colors are produced by other minerals that came in contact with the quartz during its formation. These different minerals produce the crystal's particular energetic healing frequency.

These frequencies, which can be organized largely along the lines of their color, impart that vibration to you, the healer, or your subject whenever you work with them. Therefore, when you want to heal a particular chakra center or its related organs, use the appropriate stone.

It is over-simplifying to say that each chakra is associated with a single color, however, it is necessary to make this generalization in your early study.

A more complete description of the chakras and their colors is given by Annie Besant and C. W. Leadbeater in the book, *Thought-forms*, which illustrates their various colors with colorful illustrated plates. When purchasing this book, be sure to get the version that contains the color-illustrated plates, as there is one in publication that does not. Another very good reference is the book, *Intermediate Studies of the Human Aura*, by Djwal Kul.

But, for now, you should understand that lower chakras are considered to be more substantial. These are the ones that govern our physical energy and our physical reproduction. They are associated with heavier, darker colors such as red, dark red and orange.

As you proceed up the body, the chakra system becomes increasingly emotional, mental and, finally, spiritual in nature.

The solar plexus and the heart are associated with emotions of fear and love. Their colors are orange and green, respectively. Their associated organs help keep the body working with their digestion and the pumping of blood. The solar plexus is, also, the seat of emotional instinct or intuition or the lower psychic center.

The throat chakra and the third eye chakra are associated with the colors blue and violet, respectively. These are the seats of communication both outwardly and inwardly. The throat chakra controls speech and the brain. The third eye center is the seat of the more sophisticated higher psychic center. More complex spiritual communications are received and transmitted from these two centers. It is at the third eye chakra that we receive inspiration and knowledge beyond the mundane.

The crown chakra is a shimmering white orb of light over our head that connects us with the akashic force or "All That Is."

Chakras, Colors and Gemstone Correspondences

Stones of the following colors, held in your left hand, will help you to generate the associated healing frequencies during your healing sessions and meditations, thereby, decreasing the amount of mental work you need to do. Refer to *Chapter 3* for the organs associated with each chakra center.

Base Chakra (Red): Hematite, black obsidian, black tourmaline, garnet, smoky quartz

Sacral Chakra (Orange): Orange calcite, carnelian

Solar Plexus (Yellow): Citrine, golden calcite, yellow jasper

Heart Chakra (Green or Pink): Malachite, green aventurine, rose quartz

Throat Chakra (Blue): Lapis lazuli, angelite, blue kyanite, blue calcite

Third Eye Chakra (Violet): Moonstone, amethyst, sugilite

Crown (White): Clear quartz, diamond, white calcite

If you want to impart a certain color or healing frequency to yourself, you may wear pendants or rings associated with the areas of your body in need of healing.

Lapis lazuli is a stone prized by many healers. It is good to hold or wear it when performing any type of healing because it helps you generate the healing and energetically stabilizing color blue.

ANGELA KAELIN

8

SPECIFIC MAGICAL HEALING
TREATMENTS

Whenever you are performing a healing session on yourself or someone else, begin and end with the relaxing long strokes discussed in the very first exercise of *Chapter 4*.

Although, if you have someone with a specific complaint such as a toothache, a kitchen burn or a headache, you do not need to make a ritual of things. Immediately, go to work on the specific problem.

As a general rule, problems that have not existed for a long time are easy to treat and results often come in seconds or minutes. If the pain just began a few hours ago, then it can often be relieved in a matter of seconds.

By contrast, long-standing conditions usually require longer treatments and more sessions. Examples of such conditions are chronic acne or myopia. Be patient when treating these conditions and look for gradual improvements.

Also, do not use red and orange (powerful colors of denser vibrational frequencies) on the upper organs and chakras, especially the heart and the eyes. The heart is especially delicate and it is safer to cleanse it from the back instead of the front. Orange and green are both very cleansing colors, but green is safer and more gentle. Always finish with energy tinged with blue to stabilize the work you have done.

Magical healing techniques should only be applied to pregnant women with the greatest care. They should be energized slowly and special care should be taken with regard to the lower chakras and the heart chakra not to over-energize them. Also, take great care on infants and children under the age of two, the very elderly and weak. Any treatments should be applied with the greatest gentleness and energy should be manipulated very slowly and carefully. There should be no vigorous motions when cleansing or re-energizing.

The following general treatments are given here with the standard hand movements shown in the earlier chapters. Of course, you may incorporate other methods or tools and you may, with practice, perform them entirely visually and at a distance.

Cleanse an energy center, organ or area using a counter-clockwise motion of the energy; and re-energize by using a clockwise motion.

In any of these treatments, you may generate the colors of energy you want to use in each case entirely by means of visualization or you may hold a stone of that color in your left hand. You may, also, incorporate your healing wand into these treatments.

Acne: Visualizing the color yellow or, alternatively, holding a yellow stone in your left hand, cleanse the skin with a counter-clockwise rotation, focusing on pulling out the inflammation. Do this for a few minutes, especially if it is a large area you are treating. Then, lightly re-energize with cleansing green followed by stabilizing blue.

Depending on the severity of the problem, this treatment is usually required daily or two to three times per week before improvements are obtained.

Bruises or sprains: Briefly cleanse the area with a counter-clockwise motion using the color green. Then re-energize with a clockwise motion using yellow followed by blue, if the injury is on the lower part of the body and green or violet followed by blue if it is on the upper torso or head region.

Burns: In the case of minor burns, pull the depleted energy out using the color green. Visualize a greenish white light emanating from your right hand and make a counter-clockwise rotating motion. Do not re-energize, immediately because this may cause the pain to return. If you make this mistake, simply pull the energy out again, using the counter-clockwise motion.

Constipation: Hold a reddish or orange stone (associated with the base or sacral chakras) in your left hand or visualize a white light tinged with dark red or orange. Begin by cleansing the area of the lower abdomen with your hand rotating in a counter-clockwise motion while visualizing a projection of orange-tinged energy coming from your fingers and palm. Do this for a matter of seconds or minutes. A few minutes of this movement and visualization should produce a bowel movement.

This is usually extremely effective. You may, also, speak to the intelligence of the bowels and tell them to "relax."

Afterward, re-energize the area with blue-tinged energy.

Cuts, abrasions and puncture wounds: Once the bleeding has stopped, speed the healing of these wounds by using a counter-clockwise motion while visualizing a healing and cooling green light to cleanse the area and reduce inflammation. Afterward, re-energize the area using a clockwise motion, first using green, then finishing with stabilizing blue. You may alternate these treatments, finishing by energizing the area.

Depression: (See the healing protocol for *Relief of Extreme Fatigue*, below.)

Diarrhea: Mentally instruct the digestive system to slow down. Cleanse lightly with green, then re-energize with green followed by blue.

Ear Problems: Cleanse and re-energize the energy centers of each ear with green. Green can be helpful in cases involving infection. Any time there is pain, there may be infection. Incidentally, this is the energetic principle upon which ear candles work; they are a passive tool to pull the depleted and diseased energy out.

Eye Problems, including Myopia and Presbyopia: Cleanse the eyes by energizing the third eye chakra and the two minor chakras located at each temple. Remove depleted energy and congestion. Then, re-energize using green followed by blue. Use small, short movements for these small, delicate organs and do not cleanse or energize vigorously, but very slowly and gently.

Fatigue, Extreme: (See the healing protocol for *Relief of Extreme Fatigue*, below.)

Female Problems: Speak to the organs and tell them

what they are to do according to the particular problems. For example, you may command the organs to become stronger and firmer. If there is too great a flux, speak to the organs and say, "Slow down! Cease!"

Magnetize fallen or prolapsed organs with your hands, moving them back into place. Gently, command weakened muscles to become stronger.

Alternate, cleansing and energizing motions until pain is alleviated.

Headache: Different kinds of headaches require different treatments.

To treat a sinus headache, stand behind the subject, visually reach into the congested area and pull the energy out using the color green. This can be accomplished in a matter of seconds. You will know you have succeeded when clogged sinuses suddenly begin to drain. At this point, the subject may begin to feel slightly nauseous. A small meal or a slice of bread should quell the nausea. Also, try a few drops of pure, food grade, peppermint essential oil on the tongue or inhaled on a tissue. (See the procedure for *Relief of Sinus Headache* below.)

Headaches caused by tension may respond to cleansing followed by re-energizing using green and blue energy. You may have to repeat this process a few times to see results. If sore muscles in the neck and back are concerned, these should also be cleansed and re-energized.

Heart: Treat the heart from the back and do not cleanse or re-energize with too great a vigor. Since there are multiple components to the heart and different possibilities of imbalances, you should use your pendulum or your intuition to determine exactly how to apply your treatment. Often heart pain responds quickly to a gentle re-energization with the color green, performed from the back of the heart chakra.

Generally, you should cleanse and re-energize this organ using white light tinged with green and violet, finishing with stabilizing blue.

The heart is an intelligent organ, so speak to its intelligence. Ask it to tell you how you can help it. Remind it that is must be quiet, calm and regular in its action.

Some ailments of the heart are cause by trauma or sorrow. In such cases, give the heart permission to heal itself. Tell it, "You have suffered long enough now. It is time for you to be strong and steady, again."

Indigestion: Energetically cleanse the stomach using green and yellow. Re-energize with white energy tinged with green. Green is very cleansing, but much more gentle than the denser, lower chakra colors, red and orange.

Speak to the intelligence of the stomach and address the apparent problem. For example, say, "You must relieve the congestion and inactivity. You must act with life and energy. Wake up! You must now become strong, healthy and active. You have an important job to do. From now on, digest food properly and nourish the whole body." Again, speak to the mind of the organ, not the mind of the patient.

Do this treatment five to ten minutes daily or as necessary.

Insomnia: Perform long sweeps over the body using violet or blue.

Kidneys: Cleanse the organ alternating green and orange. Then, energize with green, orange and finally blue.

You may have to repeat the sequence of cleansing and energizing to achieve results.

Liver: Cleanse the liver with orange and yellow followed by green. Re-energize with orange and yellow. Finally, stabilize the energy of the organ with blue.

Speak to the liver. "Liver, from now on you will act properly. You will secrete the proper amount of bile, no more and no less. You will let it flow freely and perform its job."

Male Problems: For a swollen prostate gland, cleanse the area with orange and green. Slowly, re-energize with blue energy. Don't overdo it.

In cases of impotence, begin by sweeping the area with orange. Then re-energize with orange, even dark orange or red can be used. Stabilize this energy by applying a small amount of blue energy.

Skin rashes: Treat these as you would acne. In acute cases, the treatment time should be much shorter.

Toothaches: Remove the dirty depleted energy from the painful area with one or two fingers using the counter-clockwise motion and the color green. This might be the only treatment necessary.

If pain persists, energize the area with green and blue. Cleanse it, again, with green. Then, with a steady projection from your fingers or your wand, apply blue-tinged energy to the affected area.

There is no limit to the kinds of illness, discomfort or infection that can be alleviated by manipulating the vital force.

Almost every treatment involves the use of color, most often blue, cleansing and removing depleted or congested energy and re-energizing with healthy vital force. When you treat yourself or someone else successfully make a note in a special notebook or journal so you will remember what worked on what specific condition.

You will learn a great deal by applying healing techniques to yourself and using them on other people whenever the opportunity arises.

Healing Yourself

You can heal yourself by applying magical healing techniques directly to your own body while sitting, standing or reclining. When you perform the clockwise and counter-clockwise motions on yourself, do it as if you were facing yourself.

To balance your chakras through visualization, go somewhere you can relax undisturbed by noises or other interruptions. Imagine vital energy entering your two lower chakra centers. These are swirling vortices of white energy tinged with red. Visualize this for about a minute. Then imagine this energy working its way up from one center to another, changing its color from red to orange, yellow, green, blue, violet and finally pure shimmering white at the crown chakra, thus re-vitalizing all of them.

An extremely effective way to treat yourself and practice the same skill required in treating anyone at a distance is to astrally project. This is not as difficult as it sounds. Again, recline and relax. Just as you saw yourself lifting out of your body in *Chapter 5, Breathing Exercise for Increased Energy and Wisdom*, allow yourself, by means of visualization, to actually leave your physical body lying at rest where it is. Then, step behind your physical self and administer the healing treatment to your own body just as you would to another person. You may visualize yourself going through the motions of cleansing organs, cells and energy centers and re-energizing them.

Performing magical healing on yourself is one of the best ways to learn what really works and how well it works. For instance, whenever you are working on yourself and the motions you are using produce any discomfort or pain, stop and change what you are doing. This is how you learn for yourself the effects that the motions have, for example, how vigorously to energize and when to stop or do something completely different.

The following are two difficult cases a healer may face in self-healing. The first involves a more direct healing on the body and the second an instance of astral projection.

Relief of Sinus Headache

While a healer can easily relieve them for others, headaches of any kind can be a serious obstacle for the self-healer because the intense pain can make it very difficult for the healer to focus his or her energy for more than a few seconds. Sinus headaches can be extremely painful and difficult to treat with pain killers and many sinus medications have unpleasant side effects. Moreover, even after you have removed yourself from the source of the allergen, the pain and pressure of a sinus headache may continue for a few days.

Sinus pain is caused when the membranes of the sinus passages become irritated. The body releases mucous as a protective measure, but it is this build up of pressure that causes excruciating pain and swelling in the head, in the face, especially around the eyes, and sometimes in the jaws and the nerves of the teeth.

The following procedure illustrates how to relieve your own sinus headache pain:

After you have removed yourself from the source of the allergic response, lie very still for a few minutes so that the pressure and pain settle into an area of your head that you can identify. Locate the source of the worst pain and pressure. Then, go into a meditative state.

Visualize the mass of unwholesome energy at the site of the pain, then, raise your hand to this location and rotate your fingers in a counter-clockwise direction, spiraling outward from this spot. If you visualize a color to this energy, it should be light green for its delicate, cleansing power. See the mass of energy coming out of this location and forming a mass outside your body. The mass of energy may seem a little sticky, so pull a large mass of this energy out away from you before visualizing it being disintegrated in flames. If necessary, repeat this procedure, again, until you feel the mass of physical congestion in your sinus cavity disperse and move down and out of your body. If you have more than one area of sinus blockage, treat those areas, as well.

Sinus drainage can cause mild nausea, so be prepared for this with food grade peppermint oil, which you can sniff and perhaps place one or two drops on your tongue to relieve it.

If you do the above exercise properly, you will experience complete drainage in a matter of minutes. As with all magical healing procedures, you must mentally connect with the subtle energy of the physical mass causing the blockage. When you remove the subtle energy, the physical mass itself will be released and recovery from your sinus headache will follow very swiftly. With practice, this operation can be performed entirely mentally and the need for hand motions eliminated.

Relief of Extreme Fatigue: Restoration of the Vital Force After a Shock or Prolonged Stress

Trauma, severe injury, serious illness and prolonged chronic stress can lead to extreme fatigue. A person can become easily tired and even a good, long sleep does nothing to re-energize the body. This can lead to a feeling of weakness in the legs and an overall sense of loss of physical strength.

Metaphysically, what is going on is that major and minor chakra centers in the lower torso are not functioning well and the body is not taking in enough vital force. Physically, there may be adrenal fatigue, a condition not generally recognized by allopaths, but which is, nonetheless, very real. Allopaths frequently misdiagnose this condition as a mental disorder (depression), when it actual has a very physical cause.

A case like this presents an obstacle to a healer because not only does their own life force becomes so low that it is difficult to perform day to day tasks, it makes the act of healing others nearly impossible. But, you can use magical healing to remedy the problem very quickly with the following procedure:

Caution: Do not perform this procedure on pregnant women or infants.

To restore and maintain the body's life force supply, lie comfortably on your right side. Visualize the following three centers: The back navel chakra, located behind the navel on the spinal column; the root chakra, which is located on the perineum; and the spleen chakra, a minor center located at this organ, which lies to the upper left of your stomach.

Begin by lying comfortably on your right side. Go into a light trance and visualize your astral body lifting out, away from your physical body. Optionally, visualize only the astral energy of your hands lifting out of your physical body and placing themselves behind your back at the rear of your navel chakra.

If your psychic sight is good, you may see a large cord attached here going to some unknown place. This is an energy attachment, which is draining your body. Whether you see it or not, make a hacking motion with your astral hands across this center to sever any astral cord that might be there.

At the back navel chakra, using a counter-clockwise motion with your astral hands, remove a small amount of energy from this energy center. Do this for only a few seconds. Then, stop and begin circling your astral hands in the opposite direction to energize the chakra center with a very dense energy, much denser, than you would use on any upper body chakras. See this energy as mostly yellow, tinged with dark red and orange. These are the colors of the base, sacral and solar plexus chakras of the lower body.

As you continue to energize the back navel chakra, see this energy center on your back, which may appear very small, widening to a diameter of about three to four inches (7.5 to 10 cm). Do not widen it much further than this because to do so can cause a tightness in the chest and hypertension. Continue to energize this center, seeing copious amounts of this dense energy flowing in. This is a very powerful energy center, so you may actually feel a surge of energy rushing into your body. Temper the flow, however, and don't overdo it. Bring the energy in steadily until the center will not accept anymore.

After you have done this, turn your attention to the base chakra on the perineum. Energize this center with your astral hands, using a clockwise motion and visualizing a white light, densely tinged with red. Then, turn to the spleen, where there is a minor chakra center. Energize this center with yellow and orange.

Then, energize each of the these three centers you have just worked on with white light tinged with blue to stabilize the work you have done.

Afterward, balance the chakra centers as previously discussed. You will likely feel a remarkable difference in your energy level and the strength in your legs. Continue this operation each day until you no longer perceive a weakness, your extreme fatigue is gone and you feel like your old self, again.

This condition of extreme fatigue is a very serious one for healers or anyone else. Dietary support includes fresh onions and garlic. (Take caution with onions if you are taking pharmaceutical blood thinners because they naturally possess this property. Consult your physician before making any dietary changes.) If you suspect an energy drain is occurring, wear a bright red cord tied around your waist, wrist or neck, to protect and maintain your personal life force supply.

SPIRIT COMMUNICATION AND AIDE

During the course of conducting any aspect of magical healing, while you are learning, exercising your intuition or actually performing a healing, you may call upon spirits to help you.

Much like a magical tool, this is another way to relieve yourself of some of the pressure of using your own vital force and your own abilities.

You may invoke the aide of healing angels, either your own guardian angel or call upon Raphael, Uriel or Chamuel by name. Ask them to bless your work, increase your personal power, knowledge and abilities to heal yourself and others.

Call upon the aide of spirits who were healers during their lifetimes. Groups of people conduct regular seances to request advice from healing spirits. Individuals can do the same thing. Be open to different methods of spirit communication through which you may receive instruction, inspiration and healing power.

Ask spirits to use you as a channel for their healing abilities. Ask to be spoken to in dreams. Ask for inspiration and for direct, conscious communication from these spirits through automatic writing or digital recordings. Very strong, enlightened spirits can communicate with receptive, calm-minded people in very physical ways, if they are given the opportunity.

Whenever you perform healing magic for another person, ask for help and guidance from the spirits surrounding the person to be healed. Literally, you can see or sense these spirits around people. Frequently, they are grandparents, aunts or other concerned relatives. Ask them for information that would be of use in your patient's situation and for any guidance they can provide.

Pray to wise and healing saints, who displayed amazing powers during their lifetimes. Ask for their help during healings, for power, knowledge and inspiration.

St. Cyprian is the patron saint of magicians and occultists.

St. Albertus Magnus is a patron saint of healers who had great knowledge of astrology, alchemy, stones, herbs, minerals and magic.

The Virgin of San Juan is a powerful image which is associated with resurrection of the dead and the infusion of the Life Force throughout the body.

St. Barbara is associated with power of lightning and is petitioned for dynamic healing of the entire body.

Call upon an appropriate saint for each particular case, for example:

Anxiety and Nerves: St. Dymphna

Breast Cancer: St. Agatha

Cancer: St. Peregrine

Childbirth: St. Anne and St. Ramon

Eyes: St. Lucy (not only her sight, but her eyes were restored)

Fever: St. Peter

Immune System Disorders: St. Peregrine

Infertility: St. Anthony

Pregnancy: St. Augustine, St. Gerard, St. Raymond

Rheumatism: St. James

Skin: St. Peregrine

Some amazing instances of healing take place in various Christian churches. The sincere testimonies of people who claim to have been healed of all kinds of conditions, cancers and addictions cannot be reasonably discounted. These healings are sometimes performed by "the laying on of hands" (a transference of the magnetic fluid or the vital force) or by exorcism using the power of Jehovah or Jesus. The names Jehovah and Jesus are ancient words of power connected with the Hebrew Kabbalah. They are powerful when invoked, regardless of religious beliefs or lack thereof.

All of these are methods of invoking spiritual aide for healing.

Sever Ties with Spirits Who Drain the Life Force Energy

Sometimes, drains on a person's energy field can be perceived and released or cut. This is done through visualization. Not uncommonly, very sick or troubled people have energetic tentacles reaching into their bodies. Sometimes you can feel these with your hands as you are sensing for energy. At other times you can psychically see or otherwise sense them.

When you find them, make a cutting gesture in the air with your hand as if you were a woodsman cutting a piece of wood. Make this movement sharply and forcefully while visualizing the connection being severed. Sometimes a person who is grey-looking will immediately regain their natural, healthy color because they are constantly being drained.

These energy drains can come from living people, the spirits of deceased people or from demonic entities of varying degree of power and influence. In simple cases, this can be resolved in one motion. In more stubborn cases, the person must be cleansed and the spirits exorcised repeatedly to eventually reduce and finally eliminate their influence. In these latter cases, you may request help from powerful angels, the Christ, the Great Mother or the Most High.

Another powerful way to heal stubborn cases involving demonic entities is through the ceremonial magick as given in some old texts like the Lemegeton and in Israel Regardie's book, *The Golden Dawn: The Original Account of the Teachings, Rites & Ceremonies of the Hermetic Order.* These must be done by a practiced and skilled ceremonial magician to be effective. A person who is possessed by a demonic entity can be freed by calling the entity out of the person and into a magical triangle drawn upon the ground. There he is either reasoned with or vanquished by the magician.

HEALING MACHINES

Healing machines are very advanced tools that work on the basis of an esoteric science that bears a resemblance to some of the theories of quantum physics and which uses different terminology to describe the natural world than the official, conventional science. Examples of such devices include radionics machines, which use frequencies similar to radio waves, Rife Frequency generators and Hieronymus machines.

Esoteric science is a set of scientific theories about the nature of energy and matter, in which the universe is seen as being comprised of energy of infinitely dense or fine qualities, with the energy of a denser quality being associated with physical matter. This science, which pre-dates the official discovery of quantum mechanics by Werner Heisenberger, was described in great detail by his predecessors Annie Besant and Charles W. Leadbeater, although their contribution to science remains largely unacknowledged.

In esoteric science and quantum physics, the relationship between matter and energy is very strong, especially on sub-atomic levels. The tiniest pathogenic particles known are viruses. You will probably find when you begin practicing magical healing that viruses are among the easiest energies to manipulate. An magical healer can wave them away with a movement of the hands and the power of the will or use other types of energetic healing to get at them very quickly.

Both matter and energy can be measured in terms of wave frequency and speed. The wave frequencies used in magical healing are similar to radio waves, but their frequencies are lower. The idea of healing by means of such waves was first developed by Ruth Drown of Greely, Colorado in the 1920s. It was advanced by other people, most notably including Dr. Albert Abrams, Dr. Bruce Copen and Royal Raymond Rife who developed a slightly different technology, but one also based on waves.

This is a highly effective working science based on esoteric scientific theories that grew out of the work of Madame Blavatsky and the aforementioned later Theosophists, Besant and Leadbeater. It is heavily discounted and legally persecuted by the reigning scientific and medical establishments despite its efficacy.

For instance, in the U.S., you will find very few books and very little information about healing with these machines, which is called "radionics," because to discuss its practice would be to implicate yourself as a Federal lawbreaker. It is possible to obtain radionics machine and it is legal to use them to treat animals and plants in the U.S., but it is illegal to use them on human beings.

The Cadillac of all radionics machines is manufactured in England by Copen Labs, LLC. The

FDA considers these machines to be "quackery" and "fraud," so it is illegal to import them into the U.S. But, the parts can be legally imported and reassembled. Therefore, whether you live in the U.S. or the U.K, you can legally obtain one of these machines.

It works according to the same type of energy we have addressed in this book and can be used to treat the energy fields of the mental, emotional and physical body and more. If you have a basic understanding of homeopathy and the esoteric scientific theory put forth by the Theosophists, you can do what appears to be miracles to the primitive mentality of conventional, modern medical doctors.

The Hieronymus machine, which is named after its inventor, T. Galen Hieronymus, is a device similar to a radionics machine. It works to diagnose the state of matter and energy and to broadcast healing frequencies.

The Rife Frequency Generator, named after its inventor Royal Rife, is similar to the aforementioned machines. All such machines are considered "quack" devices. But, anyone who has experience with radionics knows how well it works. All such machines are, also, called psionic devices and the study and application of this science is sometimes called "psionics."

The esoteric science behind magical healing is ancient. It is impossible to know how old it is, but there are some indications in ancient manuscripts and monuments like the Great Pyramids and symbols left behind by ancient people.

Robert Pavlita was a Czechoslovakian researcher of the esoteric sciences whose discoveries were introduced to the Western world in the book, *Psychic Discoveries Behind the Iron Curtain,* by Sheila Ostrander and Lynn Schroeder, first published in 1977.

The authors were shown a variety of objects of different shapes constructed using a variety of materials, which were able to generate a magnetoelectric force. Some of these devices, which are called "Pavlita Generators," can be used to perform telekinesis or to magnetize object like paper, which cannot normally be magnetized.

These devices and the scientific theories behind them are both simple and yet very advanced. They represent the real secret of the ages that has been both hoarded and preserved by secret societies for centuries and probably millennia. At the core is the science behind the life force energy that animates all things, including those things which do not seem to be alive.

All that exists on the physical plane and any of the spiritual planes to which we, as magicians and psychics, connect ourselves, has a vibrating, binary nature. Like a battery, it is its dual nature that causes it to vibrate and to live. This esoteric scientific fact is illustrated by the Hebrew Kabbalah.

This energy can be harnessed on other levels, as well. Do not discount its power on a grand scale because it was understood by the great wizard Nikola Tesla and there are many such machines as these in use now. These include familiar technologies like cell phones and remote control devices as well as less-familiar ones, such as "earthquake machines" and "HAARP (High Frequency Active Auroral Research Program) Technology."

This energy can be used both constructively and destructively, which is why knowledge of it has been hoarded, coveted, feared and sought after. Although, the sad truth is it has been ignored by a lot of the people who could benefit humanity the most from it.

As you advance in your practice and study of this energy, the vital force, the magnetic fluid or whatever name you choose to call it by, your entire view of the world around you will broaden and expand. Because while the primary way to use and understand this force is through the medium of healing, it has many other aspects.

Having a consciousness awareness of this force in your life will ultimately give you more knowledge, strength and power.

OTHER WINTER TEMPEST BOOKS

If you enjoyed this book, you might enjoy other Winter Tempest Books:

All Natural Dental Remedies: Herbs and Home Remedies to Heal Your Teeth & Naturally Restore Tooth Enamel by Angela Kaelin

Black Magic for Dark Times: Spells of Revenge and Protection by Angela Kaelin (Fiction)

Blood and Black Roses: A Dark Bouquet of Vampires, Romance and Horror by Sophia diGregorio (Fiction)

The Forgotten: The Vampire Prince by Sophia diGregorio (Fiction)

Grimoire of Santa Muerte: Spells and Rituals of Most Holy Death, the Unofficial Saint of Mexico by Sophia diGregorio

How to Communicate with Spirits: Séances, Ouija Boards and Summoning by Angela Kaelin

How to Develop Advanced Psychic Abilities: Obtain Information about the Past, Present and Future Through Clairvoyance by Sophia diGregorio

How to Read the Tarot for Fun, Profit and Psychic Development by Angela Kaelin

How to Write Your Own Spells for Any Purpose and Make Them Work by Sophia diGregorio

Natural Remedies for Reversing Gray Hair: Nutrition and Herbs for Anti-aging and Optimum Health by Thomas W. Xander

Practical Black Magic: How to Hex and Curse Your Enemies by Sophia diGregorio

Spells for Money and Wealth by Angela Kaelin

To Conjure the Perfect Man by Sophia diGregorio (Fiction)

The Traditional Witches' Book of Love Spells by Angela Kaelin

Traditional Witches' Formulary and Potion-making Guide: Recipes for Magical Oils, Powders and Other Potions by Sophia diGregorio

ABOUT THE AUTHOR

Angela Kaelin is the author of metaphysical books, such as, *How to Communicate with Spirits: Séances, Ouija Boards and Summoning*, *The Traditional Witches' Book of Love Spells*, *Spells for Money and Wealth*, and *Magical Healing: How to Use Your Mind to Heal Yourself and Others*. She is, also, an alternative health writer and the author of *All Natural Dental Remedies: Herbs and Home Remedies to Heal Your Teeth & Naturally Restore Tooth Enamel*.

Disclaimer: The author and publisher of this guide has used her best efforts in preparing this document. The author makes no representation or warranties with respect to the accuracy, applicability, fitness or completeness of the contents of this document. The author disclaims any warranties expressed or implied. The author of this book is not a medical or legal professional and is not qualified to give medical or legal advice. Nothing in this document should be construed as medical or legal advice. The material in this book is presented for informational purposes only. The procedures described in this book should not be used a substitute for treatment from state approved, licensed medical authorities.

Nothing in this book should be construed as incitement to dangerous or illegal acts and the reader is advised to be aware of and heed all pertinent laws in his or her city, state, country or other jurisdiction. Any medical or legal questions should be addressed to the proper medical or legal authorities. The author shall in no event be held liable for any losses or damages, including but not limited to special, incidental, consequential or other damages incurred by the use of this information. Always take proper precautions with candles, sharp objects, essential oils, herbs and use only as directed.

The statements in this book have not been evaluated by any other government entity. The statements contained herein represent the legally protected opinions of the author and are presented for informational purposes only. Anyone who uses any of the information in the book does so at their own risk with the understanding that the author cannot be held responsible for the consequences.

Lightning Source UK Ltd.
Milton Keynes UK
UKHW040736020119
334844UK00001B/8/P